Made in the USA
Monee, IL
08 July 2026

56644839R00066